CAT TREATS

Delicious Homemade Treats for Happy Cats

ARTHUR FRANCES

Table of Contents

CHAPTER ONE

INTRODUCTION

Overview of Handcrafted Cat Treats

Making homemade cat treats is more than just a fun project; it's a way to make sure your cat gets the best snacks possible and benefits from healthy, customized nutrition. Making treats at home gives you complete control over the process, from choosing ingredients to combining flavors, so your cat will make the most of every bite.

Why Opt for Homemade?

1. Ingredient Control: The ability to select each ingredient that goes into making homemade cat treats is one of their greatest benefits. Homemade treats are created using premium, fresh ingredients, as opposed to commercial treats that might contain unidentified additives, fillers, and artificial preservatives. If your cat has dietary restrictions or allergies, this control is especially crucial. You can make sure that your cat's treats are not only delicious but also healthy and devoid of undesirable chemicals by choosing the ingredients yourself.

2. Steer clear of additives and preservatives: Preservatives and artificial additives are frequently used in commercial cat treats to prolong their shelf life and improve their flavor. Even though these drugs are usually safe when taken in moderation, your cat's health may not always benefit from them. By removing the need for these additives, homemade treats lower your cat's risk of developing health problems and guarantee that they are getting only natural, pure snacks.

3. Meeting Nutritional Requirements: Each cat has different nutritional requirements. Making your own treats gives you the freedom to design snacks that are tailored to your cat's particular nutritional needs. Homemade treats can be tailored to your cat's specific needs, whether they are related to food sensitivities, special diets, or medical conditions. This personalization guarantees that the treats are both healthy and safe. **4. Flavor and Freshness:** Cats tend to prefer freshly made treats over store-bought ones that may be kept for extended periods of time. Your feline friend may find the scent and flavor of homemade treats made with fresh ingredients much more alluring. This can improve the bond between you and your pet and make treat time more fun.

5. Economical Over time, homemade treats may prove to be more economical, even though there may be an initial ingredient investment. You can lower the cost per treat by making larger batches and purchasing ingredients in bulk. Because of this, homemade treats are a cost-effective choice, particularly if you frequently give your cat treats.

6. An enjoyable and imaginative activity: Creating your own cat treats can be a fun and fulfilling hobby. It makes creating treats an enjoyable endeavor by letting you try out various recipes, forms, and flavors. Making it a shared activity by involving family members can also increase the experience's creativity and enjoyment. Beginning You must become familiar with a few key components and tools before you can start creating your own cat treats. Your initial steps will also be aided by a basic understanding of basic recipes and preparation methods. This chapter will walk you through the fundamentals and give you the groundwork to make tasty and nourishing treats that your cat will adore. As we proceed, we'll look at a variety of recipes and advice to help you prepare the greatest treats for your feline companion, making sure they're not only enticing but also healthy.

The key components that your cat's food should contain

1. Superior animal protein: Cats' bodies are designed to maximize the use of animal-based proteins because they are true carnivores. The main component of your cat's diet should be a high-quality animal protein source. Good ingredients include beef, fish, turkey, and chicken. It is crucial that these ingredients appear on the food label as the first ingredient. For instance, "deboned chicken" might be the first ingredient in a premium cat food. This indicates that the most prevalent protein in the recipe is chicken. The vital amino acids your cat needs to maintain strong, healthy muscles are found in high-quality animal proteins, which also give them more energy and vitality.

2. Taurine: For cats, taurine is a necessary amino acid, and a lack of it can have detrimental effects on their health. Taurine is essential for cats' vision as well as the health of their heart, brain, and nervous system. Serious illnesses like blindness and dilated cardiomyopathy can result from its deficiency. Each serving of high-quality cat food contains a sufficient amount of taurine. Choose a food that has been enhanced with this vital nutrient by having "added taurine" listed on the label.

3. Essential fatty acids for the skin and coat: For cats to have healthy skin and a glossy coat, omega-3 and omega-6 fatty acids are necessary. These nutrients have other advantages, like lowering inflammation and enhancing cardiovascular health, in addition to making your cat look better. Ingredients like fish oil, flaxseed oil, or chicken fat are examples of high-quality foods that contain essential fatty acids. Selecting a diet high in fatty acids will benefit your cat's skin and coat health and may also lessen the quantity of hairballs they consume.

4. Vital nutrients: Minerals and vitamins are essential for maintaining your cat's health at its best. Vitamin E serves as an antioxidant, preventing cell damage, vitamin D facilitates calcium absorption, and vitamin A is vital for vision. A range of these vitamins and minerals should be present in a well-balanced, high-quality meal. For instance, to make sure your cat gets all the necessary nutrients at every meal, look for a food labeled "formula with functional ingredients."

5. The significance of staying hydrated: Cats are prone to urinary issues, and maintaining the health of their kidneys and urinary tract depends on drinking enough water. High-quality wet food is an excellent way to help your cat stay hydrated in addition to giving them fresh water. Because of its high moisture content, this kind of food may help avoid kidney stones and other urinary tract disorders. Maintaining your cat's long-term health requires that they drink plenty of water.

6. Compounds that are digestible: Some high-quality foods may contain digestible carbohydrates like rice, oats, or barley, even though cats are primarily carnivores and do not need carbohydrates in their diet. For your cat's everyday activities, these carbohydrates offer an extra energy source. A high-quality food might, for instance, include yellow peas in its recipe. Glucose, a basic energy source for energetic cats, is readily produced from these carbohydrates. Digestible carbohydrates, such as peas, can help your cat stay energetic throughout the day if they are an active cat. Because it contains fiber and other vital nutrients that enhance their diet, this ingredient may be good for your cat's health in addition to giving them energy. Maintaining your pet's general health depends on making sure the food's carbohydrate source is both high-quality and easily digestible.

7. Probiotics as well as prebiotics: The general health of your cat depends on its digestive system. To keep the bacteria in your pet's digestive tract in a healthy balance, high-quality foods may contain probiotics and prebiotics. This lowers the risk of gastrointestinal disorders and encourages effective digestion. For instance, "dried beet pulp" might be listed on a food label as a prebiotic that helps your cat's gut bacteria thrive. Rich in soluble fibers, dried beet pulp feeds probiotic bacteria and keeps your cat's intestinal microbiota in the right balance. Certain high-quality foods may also include probiotics, like Lactobacillus acidophilus, in addition to prebiotics, which will improve your cat's digestive health even more. By colonizing the intestine and aiding in the breakdown of food, these advantageous microorganisms promote appropriate nutrient absorption and help avoid problems like constipation or diarrhea.

8. Antioxidants to protect cells: By shielding your cat's cells from the harm that free radicals—which are linked to aging and a number of illnesses—cause, antioxidants are essential for maintaining their cellular health. Antioxidant-rich foods like spinach, sweet potatoes, and blueberries are recognized for their high quality. Blueberries, a natural source of antioxidants like vitamin C and flavonoids, can be included in a meal. Together, these antioxidants protect your cat's body cells, strengthening their immune system and ensuring their long-term health. This is crucial for your cat's general health because it keeps them strong and disease-resistant.

9. For food sensitivities, limited ingredients: You might choose foods with fewer ingredients if your cat has food allergies or sensitivities. These foods are less likely to cause an allergic reaction or digestive issues because they contain a small number of easily digestible ingredients. For instance, you can choose a food with a different protein source, like lamb or turkey, if your cat has a sensitivity to chicken. You can reduce the risk of digestive issues and maintain your cat's comfort and health by using fewer ingredients.

10. Steer clear of artificial coloring and preservatives: Avoiding foods with artificial colorings or preservatives is essential for your cat's best health because these additives can cause allergies, digestive issues, and other health issues, especially in sensitive cats. Rather, seek out foods that preserve the freshness of their ingredients by using natural preservatives like vitamin E (tocopherols). As with foods that use natural tocopherols, a high-quality food will take pride in not using artificial colorings or preservatives in its recipe. Some high-end foods contain natural tocopherols, which are a great way to keep your cat's food fresh without sacrificing their health. Furthermore, the integrity of natural ingredients is given priority in these premium foods, as evidenced by the list you supplied, which emphasizes natural ingredients while minimizing the use of artificial additives to guarantee your pet receives the best possible nutrition. For your cat's long-term health and wellbeing, you must feed them a high-quality, well-balanced diet. You can ensure your beloved feline companion receives the best nutritional care possible by carefully selecting foods that meet these ten criteria, which will invest in their longevity and vitality. Years of happy and healthy company will be your cat's way of saying "thank you."

CHAPTER TWO

STEPS IN MAKING CAT TREATS

Make Your Own Tuna Cat Treats

I can't wait to show you this homemade cat treat recipe. Introducing my homemade tuna cat treats, which are naturally grain, gluten, and dairy free, and only take a few minutes to prepare.

Grain-Free Tuna Cat Treats Made at Home

Ingredients

1 egg

1 tin tuna (about 120g/4oz) in spring water (not brine) that has been completely drained

Recipe

1. Line a baking sheet with baking parchment or greaseproof paper and preheat the oven to 170C (330F).

2. Separate the white from the yolk by cracking open the egg. Put the white in a large mixing bowl and discard the yolk.

3. Beat the egg white with a hand whisk or an electric whisk until it forms stiff peaks when the whisk is removed. Put aside.

4. Pour the tuna can into the blender's bowl (I find a small blender is ideal for this). Stir the tuna into 2 tablespoons of the whisked egg white until the mixture is a smooth paste with no lumps or flakes.

5. Take the tuna paste mixture out of the blender with a spatula, then gently fold it into the remaining egg white that has been whisked. When mixing the two, be careful not to remove too much air from the mixture.

6. Pour the resultant mixture into a piping bag fitted with a tiny star nozzle. Line the baking sheet with parchment paper and pipe the mixture into small rounds. Avoid making the swirls too big because that would make it difficult for your cat to consume the treats.

7. The treats should be dry to the touch and easily removable from the baking parchment after 20 to 25 minutes in the oven. After transferring to a wire rack to cool, store in airtight jars. They can be stored for up to 2 weeks if kept dry and cool. When the nuggets of tuna-ey goodness are taken out of the oven and allowed to cool completely, they actually become a little harder. As a shameful admission, the end product is a crunchy tuna snack that is so delicious. Although they are a bit too dry for most people's palates, I have the unshakeable impression that they

would make the ideal savory bar snack to go with a dry martini. Keep it a secret. Remember that these are still treats, so your cat's regular diet shouldn't be replaced by them. Your cat will quickly realize that they must have been very good when they receive one if you treat them like the treats they are.

Recipe for Chicken and Pumpkin Bites

This easy and healthy recipe gives your cat a tasty, high-protein, high-fiber treat by combining cooked chicken and pumpkin.

Here's how to make these delicious morsels:

Components:

- 1 cup of cooked chicken, either finely chopped or shredded

- 1/2 cup of canned pumpkin (pure pumpkin, not pumpkin pie filling)

- 1/4 cup oat flour (or, in the event that oat flour is not available, regular flour)

- 1 egg

- 1 tablespoon of low-sodium chicken broth (optional; adds flavor) • 1/2 teaspoon of dried catnip, if desired for visual appeal

Tools:

- A bowl for mixing

- A blender or food processor (optional, for a finer consistency)

- A rolling pin

- Optional cookie cutters for shaping

- A baking sheet

- A baking mat made of silicone or parchment paper

- A cooling rack

Guidelines:

1.Preheat Oven: Set the oven's temperature to 350°F (175°C).

2.Prepare the chicken by cooking and shredding it, if you haven't already. It can be cooked through by baking, boiling, or sautéing, then allowed to cool before being finely chopped or shredded.

3.Combine Ingredients: Put the chicken broth, oat flour, canned pumpkin, shredded chicken, and egg in a mixing bowl. Add dried catnip to the mixture as well, if using. Until all the ingredients are well combined, thoroughly mix. It should be manageable but a little sticky.

Note: You can pulse the ingredients in a blender or food processor until thoroughly mixed if you'd like a smoother texture.

4.Roll Out Dough: Use a rolling pin to roll out the dough to a thickness of approximately 1/4 inch after lightly flouring a clean surface. You can add a little more flour on top if the dough is too sticky.

5.Cut Shapes: Cut out shapes from the dough using cookie cutters. You are free to select any shape you like, including festive shapes or tiny rounds. You can use a knife to cut the dough into tiny squares or rectangles if you don't have cookie cutters.

6.Bake: Transfer the cut-out dough pieces to a silicone baking mat or parchment paper-lined baking sheet. The treats should be firm and lightly golden after 15 to 20 minutes of baking in a preheated oven.

7.Cool: Before serving, let the treats cool fully on a cooling rack. This guarantees that your cat can safely eat them and that they are crunchy.

8.Store: Put the chilled sweets in a tightly sealed container. They can be refrigerated for extended freshness or stored at room temperature for up to a week.

Advice:

- **For More Crunch:** If you would like the treats to have more crunch, you can bake them for a few more minutes, but watch out that they don't bake too much.

- **Batch Size:** A small batch is produced by this recipe. If you want to make more treats at once, you can double or triple it.

- **Allergy Awareness:** Verify that your cat has no allergies or sensitivities to any of the ingredients.

Your cat will adore these homemade and healthful Chicken & Pumpkin Bites. Pumpkin and chicken together offer fiber and protein, which promotes your cat's general health and wellbeing. Enjoy creating these treats and seeing how much fun your cat has eating them!

Nutritious and Healthful Treats

Giving your cat wholesome treats is a great way to express your affection and promote their general health. The benefit of making your own treats is that you can keep an eye on the ingredients and steer clear of superfluous additives, so your cat will always have tasty and healthy snacks.

Here, we look at 2 outstanding recipes: Catnip Infused Treats and Salmon and Sweet Potato Chews.

Overview of Salmon and Sweet Potato Chews: 2 nutrient-dense ingredients come together in Salmon and Sweet Potato Chews to make a tasty treat that also benefits your cat's health. Omega-3 fatty acids, which are vital for preserving a healthy coat and skin, are abundant in salmon. Conversely, sweet potatoes offer essential vitamins and fiber that promote overall health and digestive well-being.

Components:

• **1 cup of cooked salmon:** Select salmon that is skinless and boneless. Omega-3 fatty acids, which are abundant in salmon, support heart health and lower inflammation. Additionally, it offers high-quality protein, which is necessary for maintaining healthy muscles and general vitality.

• **Half a cup of cooked sweet potatoes:** Rich in dietary fiber and vitamins A and C, sweet potatoes are a great food choice. These nutrients support healthy digestion and immune system function. To make blending with other ingredients easier, make sure the sweet potato is mashed.

• **1/4 cup oat flour:** Oat flour helps bind the mixture and adds a small amount of fiber. If your cat has sensitivities, it's a good substitute for wheat flour.

• **1 egg:** Offers extra protein and serves as a binder to keep the treat together.

• **1 tablespoon of optional fish oil:** Increases the treats' omega-3 content. Additionally, fish oil promotes cognitive and joint health.

• **Optional:** 1/2 teaspoon dried catnip, which adds a little taste and excitement. Catnip can encourage enrichment and play.

Tools:

• **Mixing bowl:** Used to mix the components. To blend the mixture into a smooth consistency, use a blender or food processor.

• **Rolling pin:** If desired, use this to flatten the dough.

• **Optional cookie cutters:** For cutting out interesting shapes.

• **Baking sheet:** For the chews' baking.

• To avoid sticking, use silicone baking mats or parchment paper.

• Cooling rack: To keep the sweets cold.

Guidelines:

1. Warm up the oven: Set your oven's temperature to 350°F (175°C) to start.

2. Get the ingredients ready: Make sure the salmon is cooked through before removing the skin and bones. Smoothly mash the sweet potato.

3. Mix the ingredients together: Put the cooked salmon, mashed sweet potato, egg, and oat flour in a mixing bowl. Stir thoroughly. Include dried catnip and fish oil in this step if you're adding them. Though not overly sticky, the mixture should be thoroughly mixed.

4. Blend (Selective): Blend the mixture in a blender or food processor for a smoother texture. Although it's not required, this step can help make the dough more uniform.

5. Dough Roll Out: Roll out the dough to a thickness of about 1/4 inch on a lightly floured surface. The chews are guaranteed to be crunchy and firm because of their thickness.

6. Shapes Cut: Simply use a knife to cut the dough into small squares or rectangles, or use cookie cutters to make fun shapes.

7. Cake: Place the dough pieces on a silicone baking mat or parchment paper-lined baking sheet. The chews should be firm and lightly golden after 20 to 25 minutes in the oven.

8. Calm: On a cooling rack, let the treats cool fully. This keeps them safe to store and helps them get crisp.

9. Shop: The cooled chews should be kept in an airtight container. To prolong their freshness, they can be stored in the refrigerator or at room temperature for up to a week.

Benefits

- **Omega-3 Fatty Acids:** Vital for heart health, inflammation reduction, and the health of the skin and coat.

- **Vitamins and Fiber:** These nutrients, which are found in sweet potatoes, support healthy digestion and general wellbeing.

Treats Infused with Catnip

Summary: Treats infused with catnip are a fun and engaging choice for your feline companion. These treats, which are infused with catnip, are entertaining and nutritious thanks to the addition of oat flour and eggs. Your feline friend will find treat time more interesting and pleasurable if you give them catnip because it can stimulate their mind.

Components:

- **1 cup of oat flour:** This ingredient aids in binding the treat mixture and is a good source of dietary fiber. Additionally, compared to wheat flour, it is less likely to trigger allergies.

• **Half a cup of dried catnip:** Make sure the catnip is unadulterated and unadulterated. Natural stimulation from catnip promotes excitement and play.

• **1 egg:** Offers extra protein and acts as a binder.

• **1/4 cup water:** Aids in combining the dough. For extra flavor, you can use low-sodium chicken broth instead.

• **Optional:** 1 tablespoon of olive oil can provide extra healthy fats and moisture to the dough.

• **1 tablespoon of optional dried parsley:** Enhances taste and offers slight digestive advantages.

Tools:

• **Mixing bowl:** Used to mix the components. To roll out the dough, use a rolling pin.

• **Optional cookie cutters:** For cutting out interesting shapes.

• **Baking sheet:** Used to bake the confections.

• To avoid sticking, use silicone baking mats or parchment paper.

• **Cooling rack:** To keep the sweets cold.

Guidelines:

1. **Warm up the oven:** Set the oven temperature to 175°C (350°F).

2. Mix the dry ingredients together: Put the dried catnip and oat flour in a mixing bowl. Add dried parsley to the mixture if using.

3. Include Wet Substances: Add the water (or chicken broth), olive oil, and cracked egg to the bowl. Stir until the dough starts to bind. If necessary, add more liquid to change the consistency.

4. Roll Out Dough: Roll out the dough to a thickness of about 1/4 inch after lightly flouring a clean surface. This thickness is perfect for treats that are crunchy.

5. Shapes Cut: Cut the dough into small pieces with a knife or make shapes with cookie cutters.

6. Cake: Arrange the dough pieces on a silicone baking mat or parchment paper-lined baking sheet. Bake for 15 to 20 minutes, or until golden and firm.

7. Calm: On a cooling rack, let the treats cool fully. 8. Shop: The cooled treats should be kept in an airtight container. They can be refrigerated for extended freshness or stored at room temperature for up to a week. **Benefits**

- **Catnip:** Promotes play by offering excitement and mental stimulation. • **Eggs and oat flour:** Provide vital proteins and nutrients that support general health. By adding these wholesome treats to your cat's diet, you can improve their general health and give them fun, engaging snacks. Both recipes are made with premium ingredients that will enhance your cat's health and provide mouth-watering flavor. These homemade options are sure to please your feline companion, whether it's the exciting Catnip Infused Treats or the omega-3-rich Salmon and Sweet Potato Chews.

CHAPTER THREE

TREATS FOR SPECIAL OCCASIONS AND SEASONS

A fun way to express your love and gratitude for your feline companion is to celebrate special occasions with them. In addition to making the celebrations more joyful, seasonal and special occasion treats give you a chance to give your cat tasty and nourishing snacks.

Here, we look at 2 festive recipes: Birthday Cake Treats and Holiday Tuna Wreaths.

Holiday Wreaths with Tuna Summary: Holiday Tuna Wreaths are ideal for celebrating holidays with your feline companion. Your cat's treat time will be a little more festive with these treats in the shape of festive wreaths. These tuna-filled wreaths provide a tasty and nourishing snack that is high in protein.

Components:

• **1 can of tuna in water (drained):** Essential fatty acids and premium protein can be found in abundance in tuna. To keep the treat light and nutritious, make sure it is packed in water rather than oil.

• **1/4 cup oat flour:** aids in binding the ingredients together and adds fibre. In addition, oat flour is less likely to trigger allergies than wheat flour.

• **1/4 cup grated carrot:** In addition to offering vitamins and minerals, carrots' inherent sweetness can enhance the appeal of the treats.

• **1 egg:** Offers extra protein and serves as a binder.

• **Optional:** 1 tablespoon of dried catnip, which boosts flavor and energy. • **1 tablespoon of chopped parsley (optional):** Adds taste and may help with digestion.

Tools:

• **Mixing bowl:** Used to mix the components.

• **Blender or food processor:** If necessary, to blend the mixture.

• **Rolling pin:** Used to press the dough flat.

• **Wreath-shaped cookie cutters:** For cutting out festive shapes.

• **Baking sheet:** Used to bake the confections.

• To avoid sticking, use silicone baking mats or parchment paper.

• **Cooling rack:** To keep the sweets cold.

Guidelines:

1. **Warm up the oven:** Set the oven temperature to 175°C (350°F).

2. **Get the carrots and tuna ready:** After completely draining, put the tuna in a mixing bowl. Add the grated carrot to the bowl.

3. **Mix the ingredients together:** Add the egg, oat flour, and optional ingredients such as parsley or catnip. Until the dough is well combined, mix thoroughly. To get the right consistency, add a little water if the dough is too dry.

4. **Blend (Selective):** You can blend the mixture in a food processor for a smoother consistency.

5. **Dough Roll Out:** Roll out the dough to a thickness of about 1/4 inch on a lightly floured surface.

6. **Shapes Cut:** Cut out the treats with a cookie cutter in the shape of a wreath. If you don't have a wreath cutter, you can make a wreath shape by using a round cutter and cutting out the center with a smaller

cutter. **7. Cake:** Lay the cut-out wreaths on a silicone baking mat or a baking sheet covered with parchment paper. Bake until the treats are firm and just beginning to turn golden, 15 to 20 minutes.

8. Calm: Before serving, let the treats cool fully on a cooling rack.

9. Shop: The cooled treats should be kept in an airtight container. They can be refrigerated for extended freshness or stored at room temperature for up to a week.

Benefits

• **Protein-Rich Tuna:** Offers essential fatty acids and premium protein.

• **Grated carrot:** Increases the nutritional value of the treats by adding fiber and vitamins.

Cake Treats for Birthdays Summary: A delightful way to commemorate your cat's special day is with birthday cake treats. These treats, which can be made into cupcakes or mini cakes, provide a fun and unique way to celebrate your cat's birthday. These treats are tasty and healthy because they are made with wholesome ingredients.

Components:

• **Half a cup of canned pumpkin (pure pumpkin, not pie filling):** Offers vitamins and fiber to promote overall health and digestive health.

- **1/4 cup oat flour:** Provides fiber and aids in binding the ingredients.

- **1/4 cup of turkey or chicken, finely shredded:** adds taste and protein. Make sure the meat is cooked through and deboned.

- **1 egg:** Provides protein and serves as a binder.

- **1/4 cup unsweetened plain Greek yogurt:** This protein and probiotic source gives food a creamy texture.

- **1 tablespoon of optionally chopped parsley:** Enhances taste and facilitates digestion.

Tools:

- **Mixing bowl:** Used to mix the components.

- **Cupcake molds or mini cake pans:** To form the confections. The baking sheet is used to arrange the pans.

- To avoid sticking, use silicone baking mats or parchment paper.

- Cooling rack: To keep the sweets cold.

Guidelines:

1. **Warm up the oven:** Set the oven temperature to 175°C (350°F).

2. Get the ingredients ready: Add the egg, finely shredded chicken, oat flour, and canned pumpkin to a mixing bowl. Stir until thoroughly blended.

 3. Include the yogurt: Add the plain Greek yogurt and fold gently. For added flavor, add the chopped parsley, if using.

4. Fill Molds: Transfer the mixture using a spoon into cupcake molds or mini cake pans. Use the back of a spoon or a spatula to smooth the tops. **5. Cake:** The treats should be firm and a toothpick inserted in the center should come out clean after 15 to 20 minutes of baking in the molds on a baking sheet.

6. Calm: Before taking the treats out of the molds, let them cool fully.

7. Shop: The cooled treats should be kept in an airtight container. For extended freshness, they can be stored in the refrigerator or at room temperature for a few days.

Benefits

• **Pumpkin in a can:** Offers vital vitamins and promotes digestive health. • **Turkey or chicken high in protein:** Helps maintain muscles and provides general energy.

• **Greek yogurt:** Good for digestive health, it contains protein and probiotics. These treats for special occasions and the seasons are a great way to celebrate with your feline companion. Whether it's the joyous Birthday Cake Treats or the festive Holiday Tuna Wreaths, these recipes are made with healthy, wholesome ingredients to improve your cat's health and happiness. Give your cat treats that will make them happy and healthy in addition to looking fantastic.

CHAPTER FOUR

COMMON ISSUES AND SOLUTIONS

Making homemade cat treats can be a rewarding experience, but it's not without challenges. To keep your treats looking and tasting their best, we cover common issues you might encounter, practical solutions for them, and storage and preservation tips below.

Problems and Solutions

1. Inadequate Treat Baking

The treats are either too soft or too hard, which is the issue.

Response:

• Too Soft: If the treats are coming out too soft, they might need more baking time. Verify that the oven's temperature is accurate and consistent. You can also try making the treats smaller or thinner to help them bake more evenly.

• Too Hard: If the treats are too hard, you might be baking them for too long or at too high of a temperature. Consider reducing the baking time or temperature slightly. An alternative is to add a bit more moisture to the dough, such as another egg, water, or broth.

2. Too Sticky or Dry Dough

The dough is difficult to work with because it is either too sticky or too dry.

Response:

• Too Sticky: Add more flour (whole wheat flour or oat flour) gradually until the dough is manageable. Dust your hands and the rolling pin with flour to facilitate handling.

• Too Dry: Add a little water, broth, or another egg to the dough to get the proper consistency. Mix well after each addition.

3. The Cat Has Strict Taste Preferences

Your cat is refusing to eat the homemade treats.

Response:

• Experiment with Different Ingredients: Different cats have different textures and flavors. Include foods they enjoy and introduce them to new protein sources, such as turkey, fish, or poultry.

• Introduce Gradually: If your cat is not used to homemade treats, gradually introduce them by mixing a small amount with their regular food.

• Catnip and Other Attractants: A small pinch of catnip or another favorite flavor can be added to the treats to make them more enticing.

4. Unreliable Baking

Issue: Because of uneven baking, some parts of the treats are overcooked while others are undercooked.

Response:

• Consistent Thickness: Make sure the dough is rolled out to an even thickness to promote consistent baking.

- **Turn the Baking Sheet:** Halfway through the baking time, turn the baking sheet to ensure even heat distribution.

Make sure your oven is preheated and maintained at a consistent temperature to confirm its setting. An oven thermometer can be used to verify this.

Maintaining and Storing

Proper storage is crucial to maintaining the freshness and extending the shelf life of your homemade cat treats.

The following tips will assist you in appropriately storing them:

1. Completely Cool

- **Before Storage:** Make sure the treats have completely cooled on a cooling rack before storing them. Warm treats may become soggy and possibly develop mold due to condensation from storage.

2. Utilize Airtight Containers

- **Storage Containers:** Store the treats in airtight containers to preserve their freshness. Glass jars with tight-fitting lids, resealable plastic bags, or plastic containers all work well.

- Label and Date: Indicate the type of treat and the manufacturing date on the containers to preserve freshness.

3. Refrigeration and Freezing

- Refrigeration: Homemade cat treats can be stored in the refrigerator for up to 2 weeks. This is especially beneficial for treats made with fresh ingredients like meat and fish.

- Freezing: For longer storage, consider freezing the treats. Arrange the treats in a single layer on a baking sheet and freeze until set. Next, transfer them to a freezer-safe container or resealable bag. You can keep frozen treats for up to 3 months. Thaw them at room temperature before serving.

4. Portion Size Control

- Small Batches: If you won't be using the treats all at once, store them in smaller batches. Because you only need to thaw or use what you need, the remainder stays fresher for longer.

5. Pay attention to freshness

• Check Often: Keep an eye out for mold, odd smells, or changes in texture that might point to spoiling. Throw away any treats that show these signs to keep your cat safe.

6. An appropriate environment

Treats should be stored in a cool, dry place away from heat sources and direct sunlight. This maintains their texture and prevents them from going bad. By addressing common issues and using these storage and preservation tips, you can ensure that your homemade cat treats are always safe, fresh, and enjoyable for your feline friend. A great way to provide your cat with nutritious snacks that meet their dietary needs and preferences is to make your own treats.

THE END

www.ingramcontent.com/pod-product-compliance
Lightning Source LLC
Chambersburg PA
CBHW081637250726
48657CB00009B/2932